r Lungs

Approach to the
 piratory System

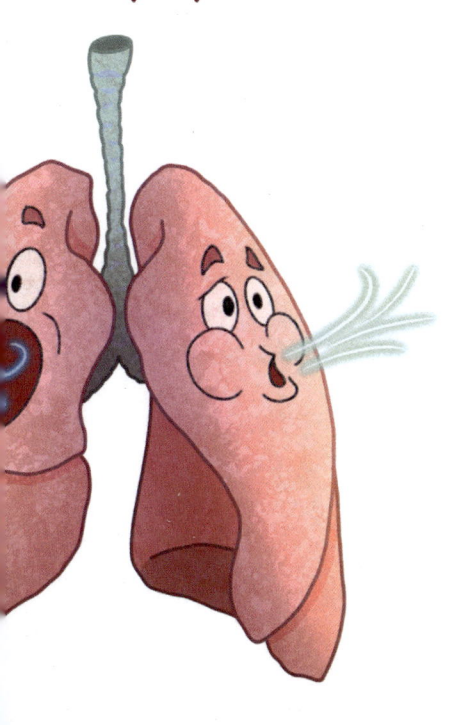

 n by Dr. McCann
 d by Quintin McCann

 ody McCannics

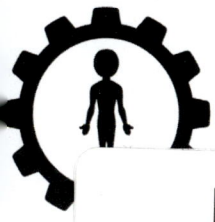

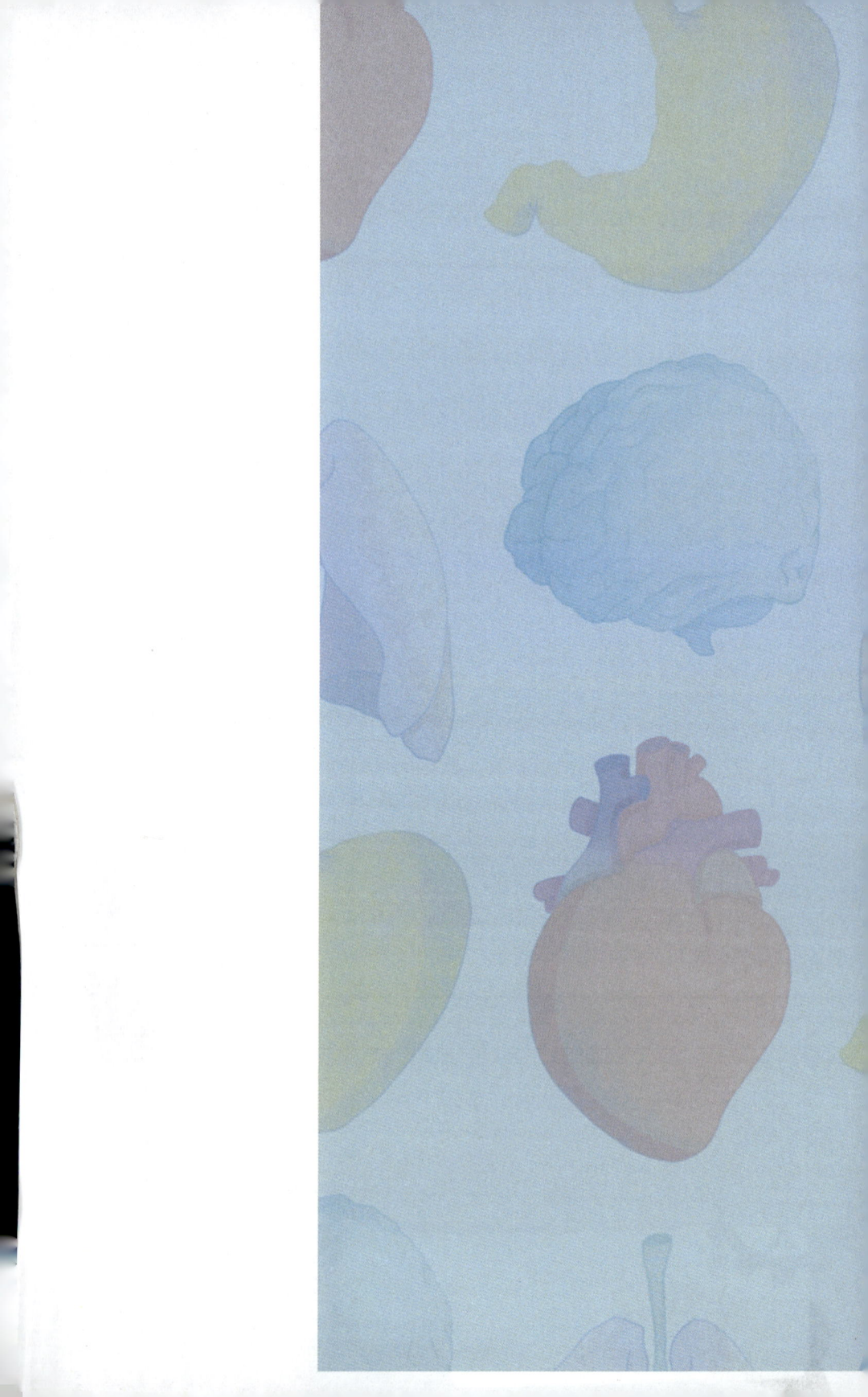

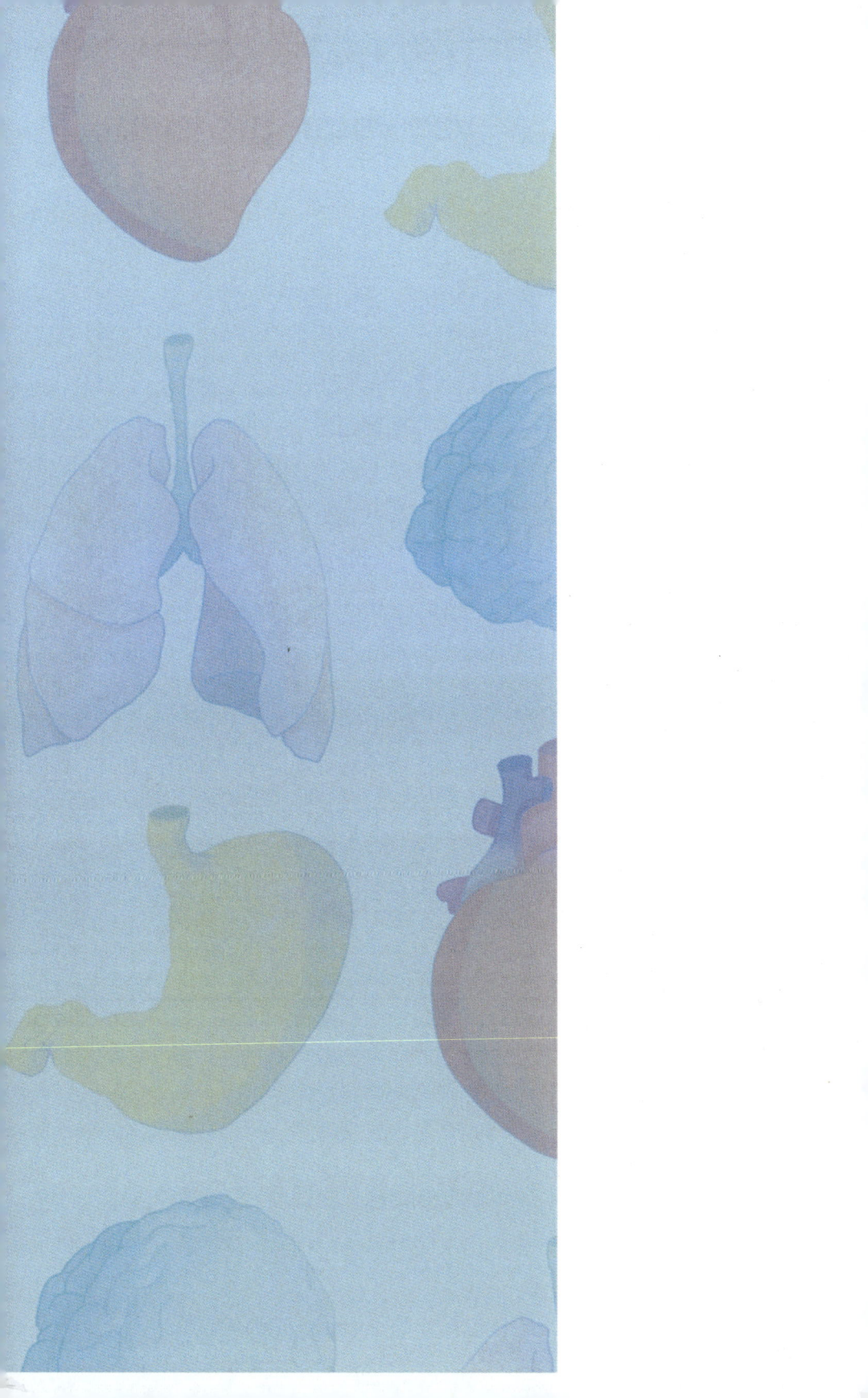

Hey there pal,
yes you right there.

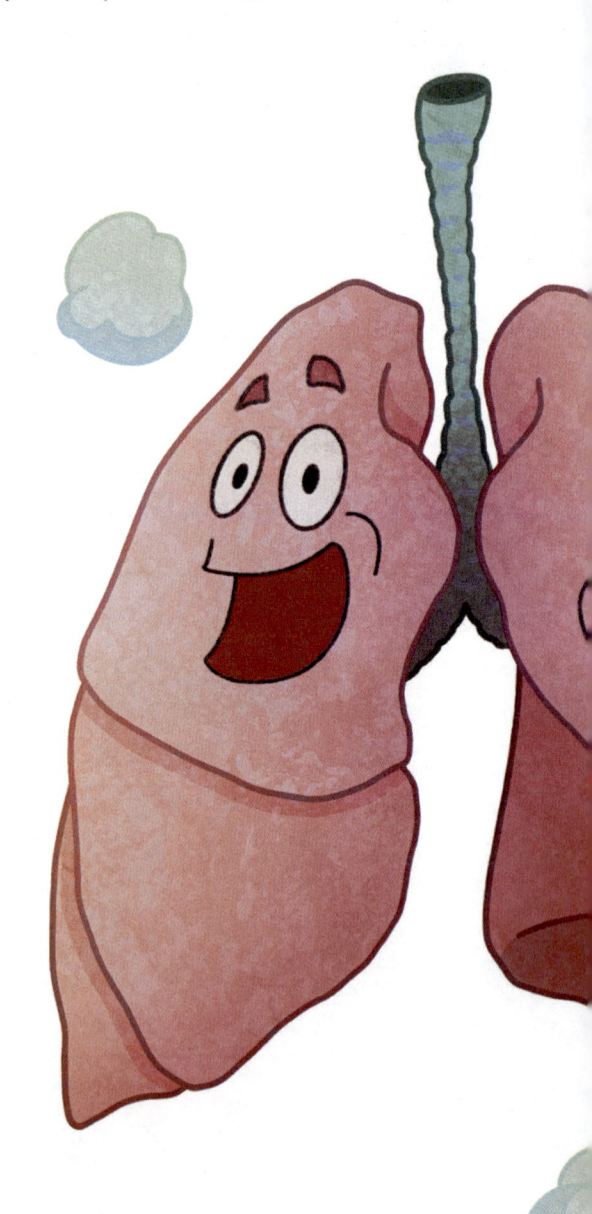

We're **Your Lungs**
and we like air.

reath in

eath out

ve tell you what
all about.

We fill up with air next to your heart.

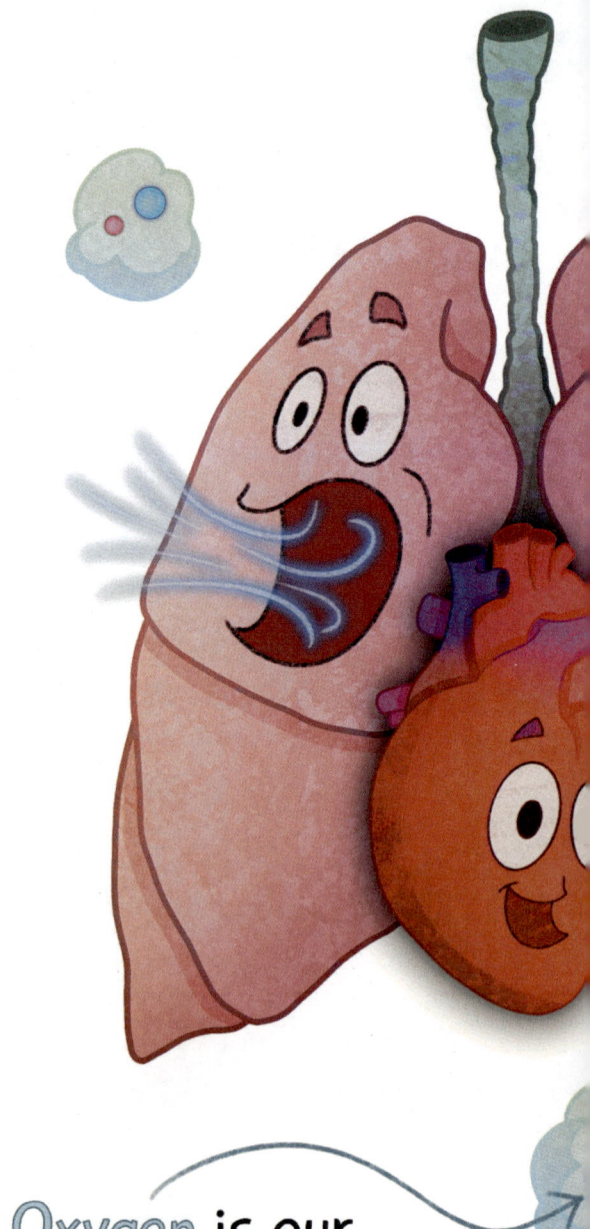

Oxygen is our favorite part.

ir in
mouth or nose,

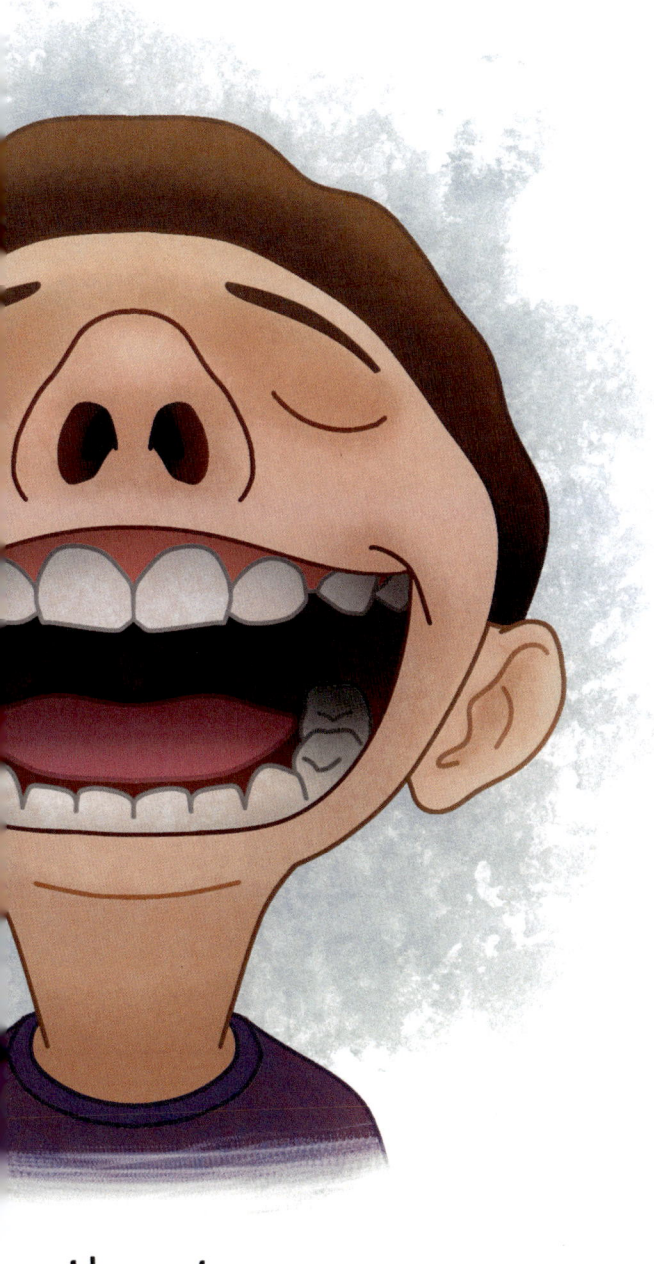

ur throat
ows.

The air then finds tunnels one and two.

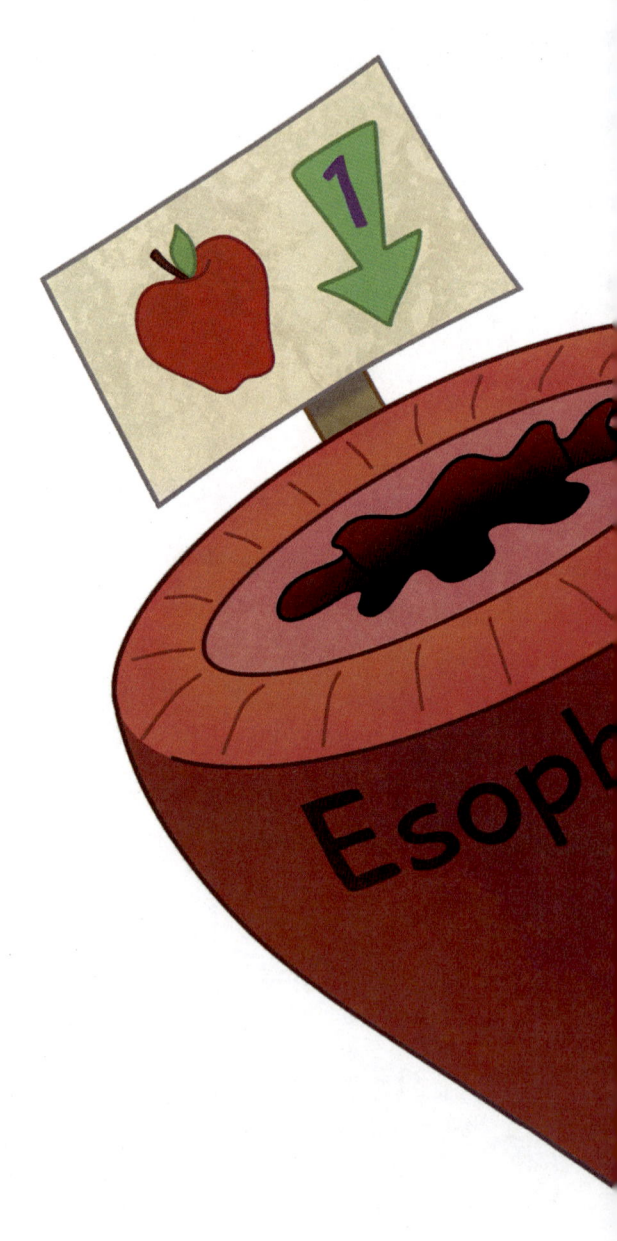

It skips the first- that's for the food you

the trachea,
some say.

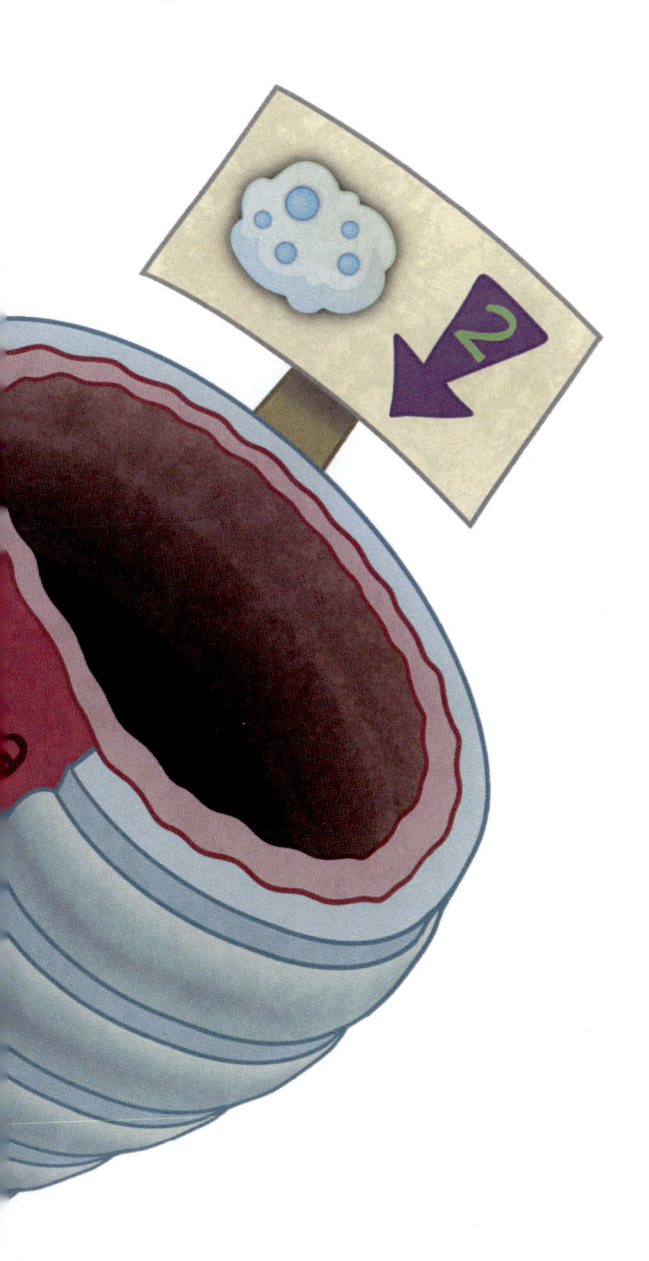

Air enters here
and continues on its way.

Down the trachea
splitting left and right,

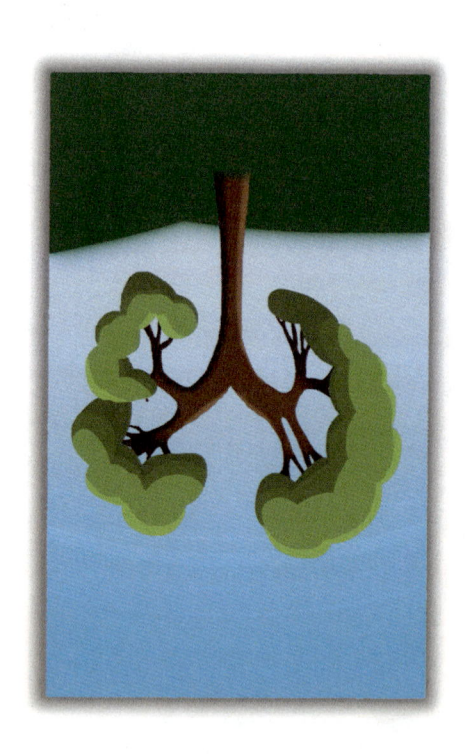

and like a tree
that's not upright,

split up

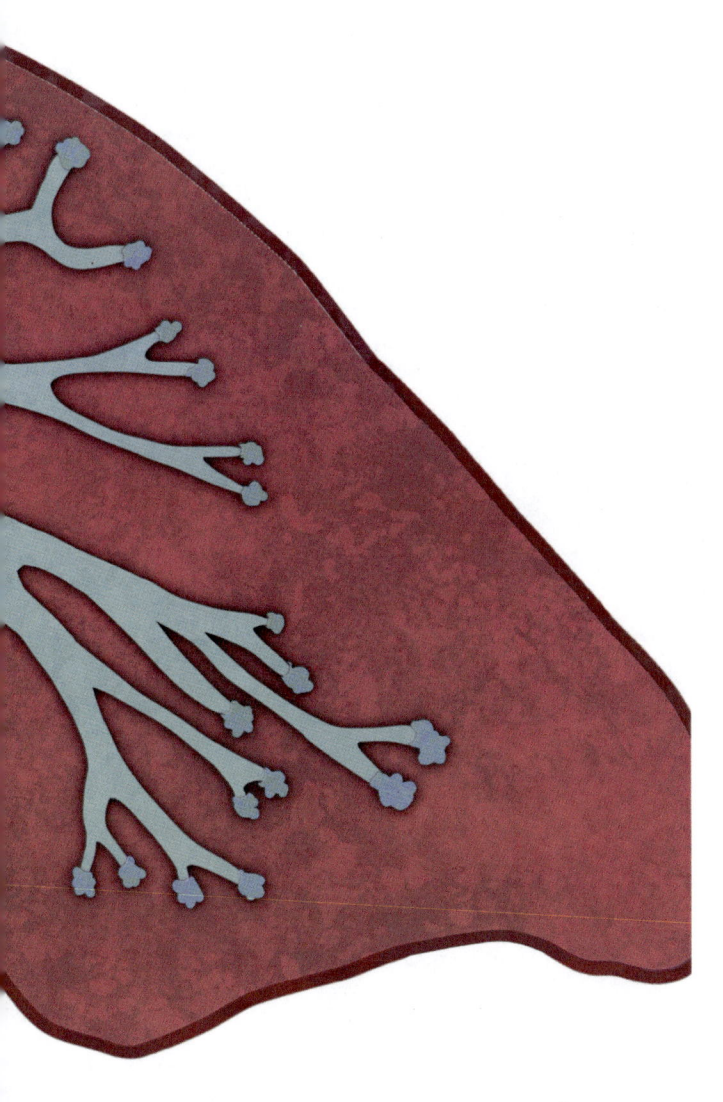

e,

branches called bronchi.
airways galore!

At the end of each of t
thousands of branches

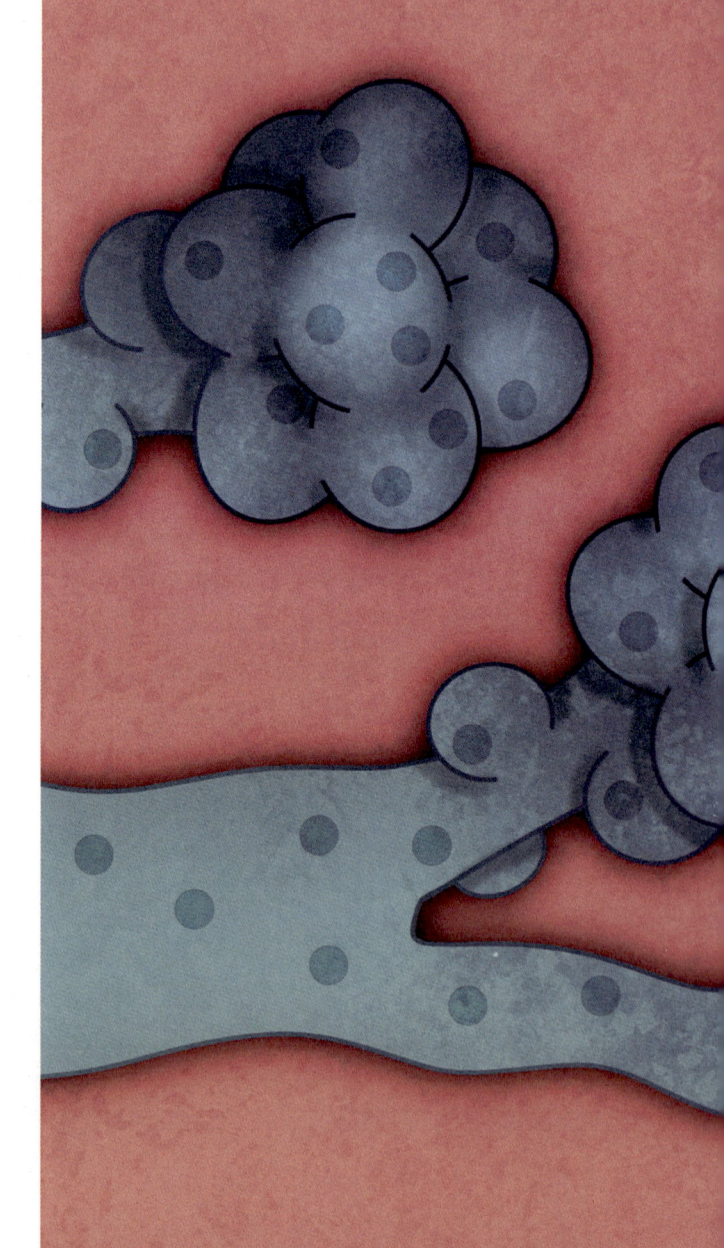

is a bunch of small sacs
filled with air that it cat

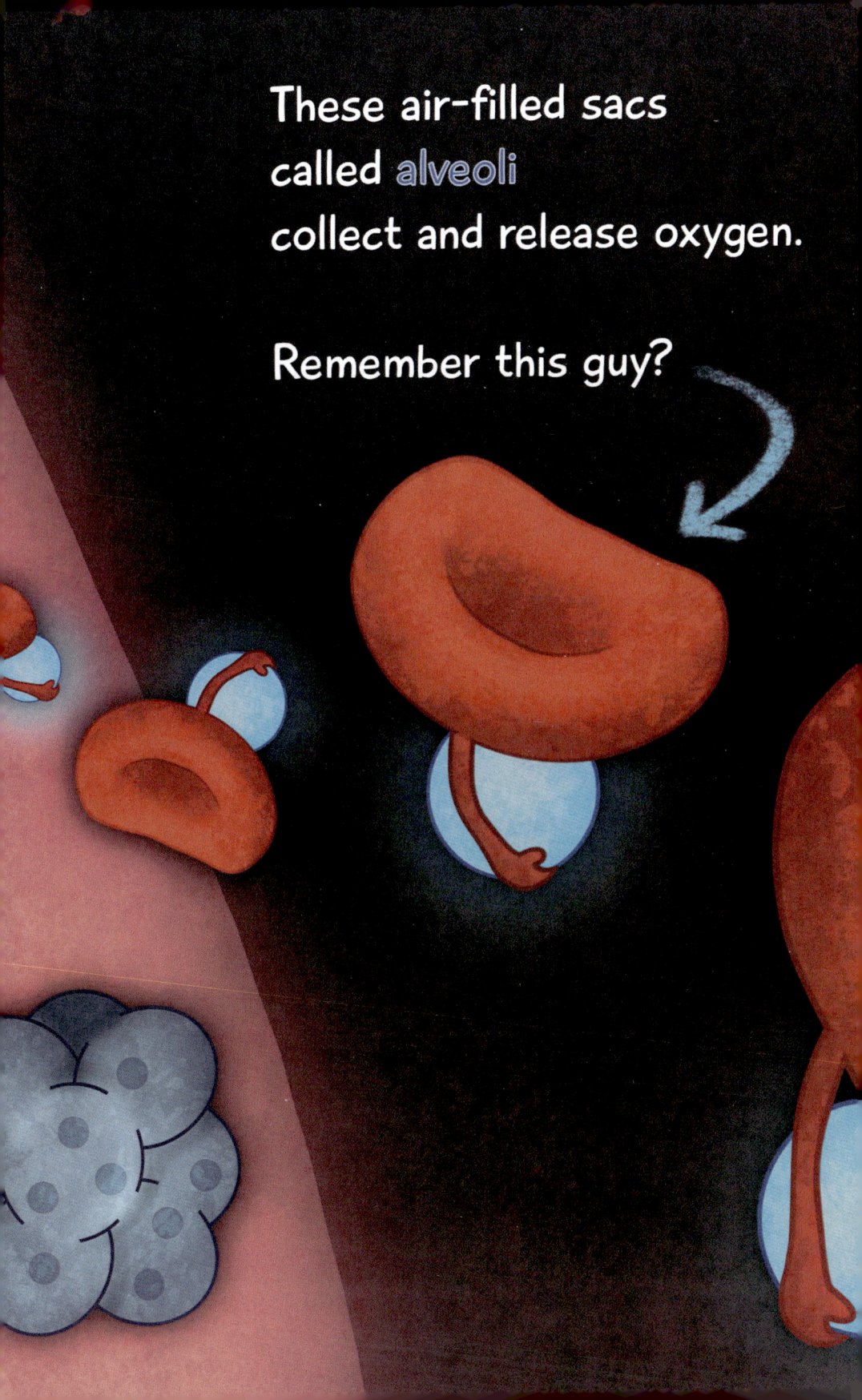

These air-filled sacs called alveoli collect and release oxygen.

Remember this guy?

For the cells in your body to make energy,

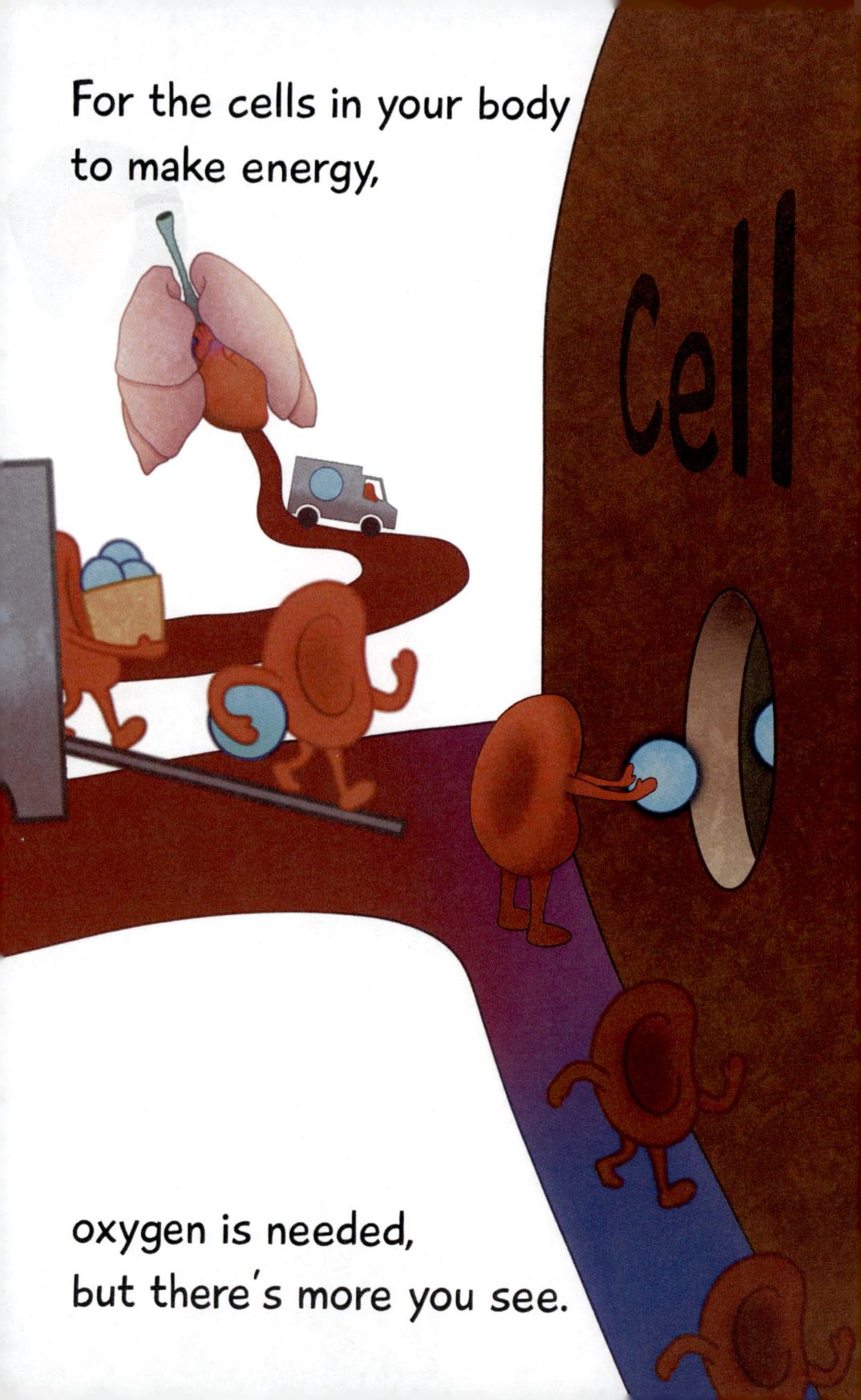

Cell

oxygen is needed,
but there's more you see.

Add food from your stomach (like apples and cheese),

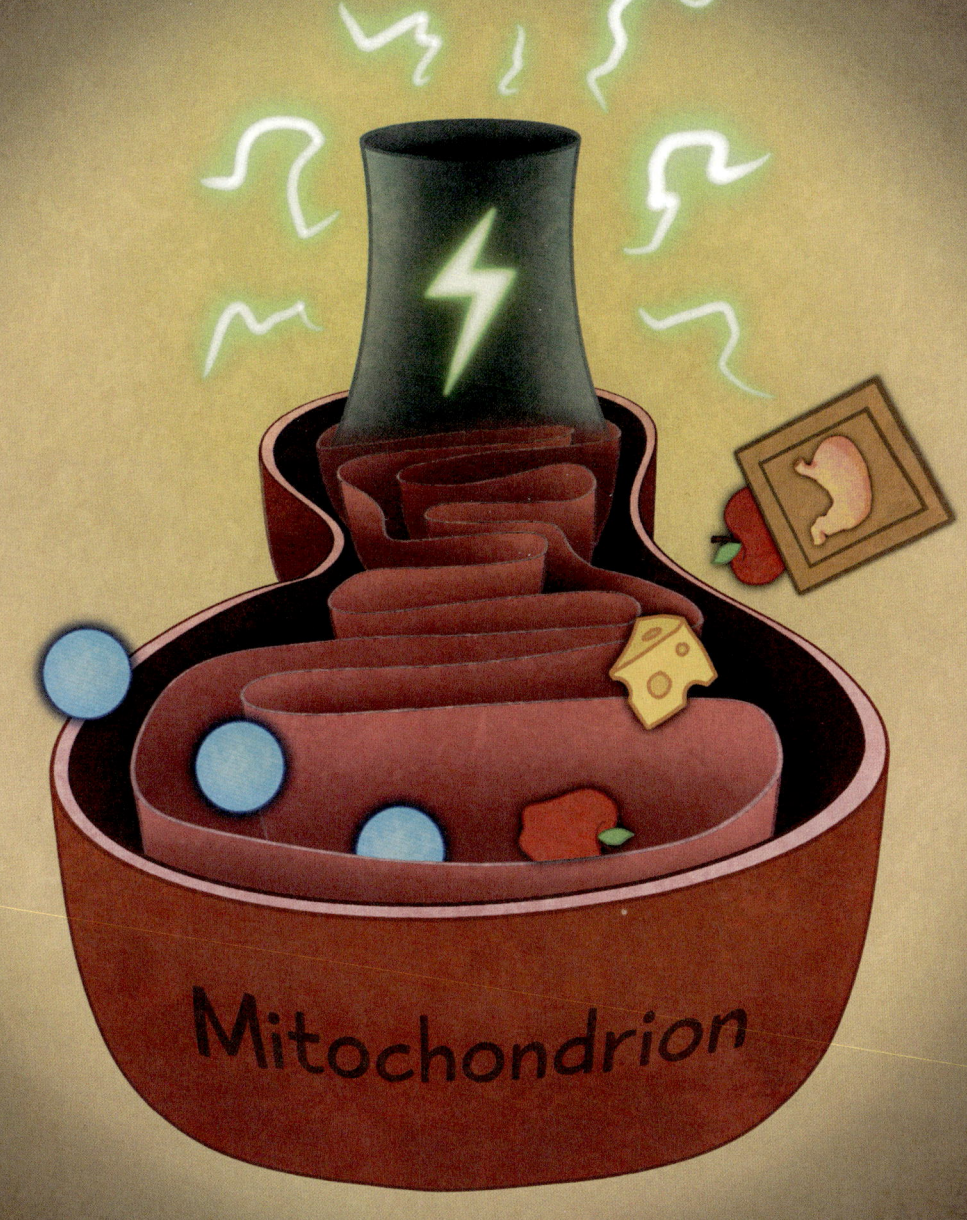

Mitochondrion

then energy gets made to use as you please.

During this process,
a by-product is made.

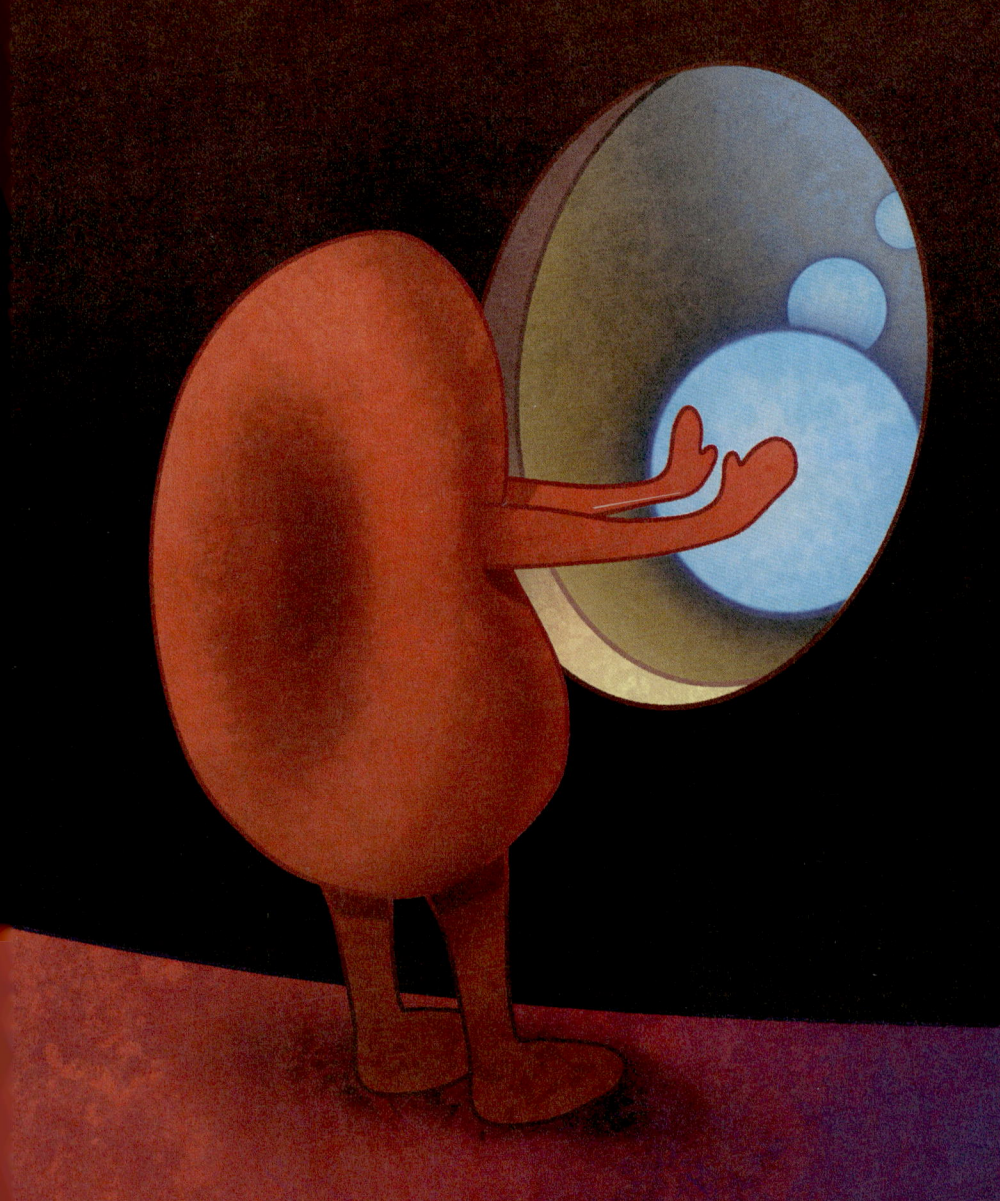

Carbon dioxide.
It's time for a trade.

CO_2 for O_2,
in this situation,

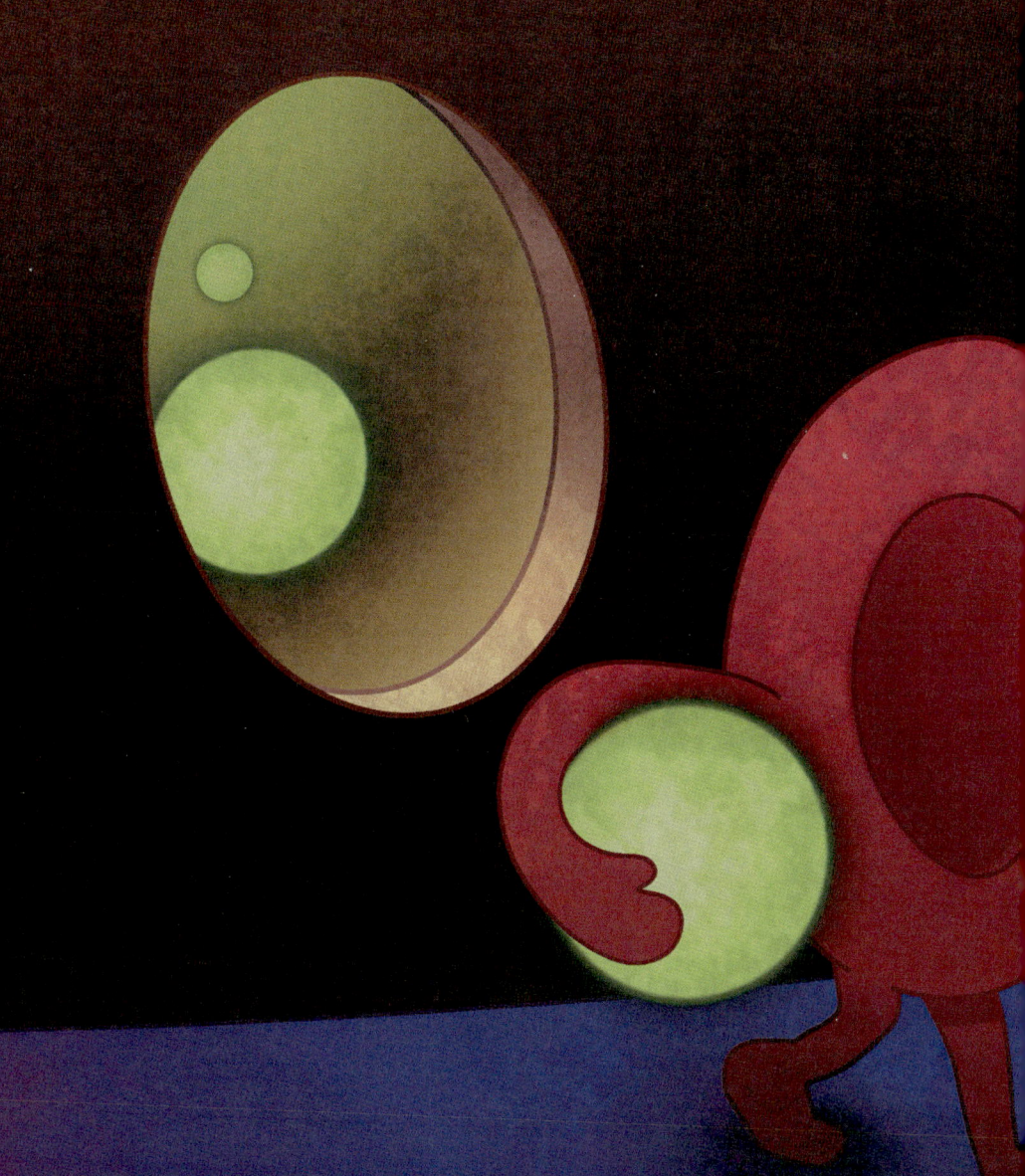

the exchange of the gases
is called respiration.

Then back to your lungs,
CO_2 takes a ride.

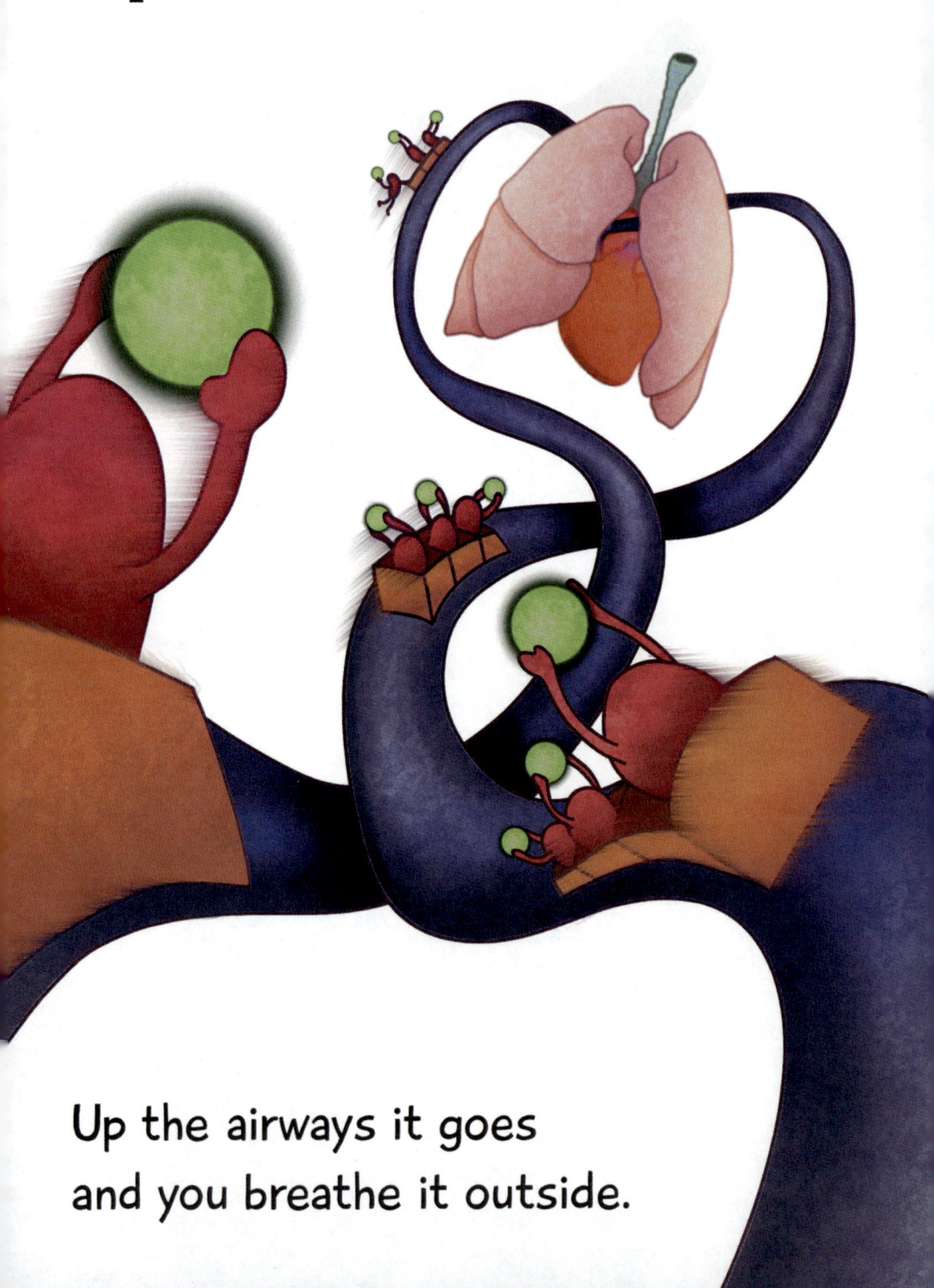

Up the airways it goes
and you breathe it outside.

This movement of air, for our conversation,

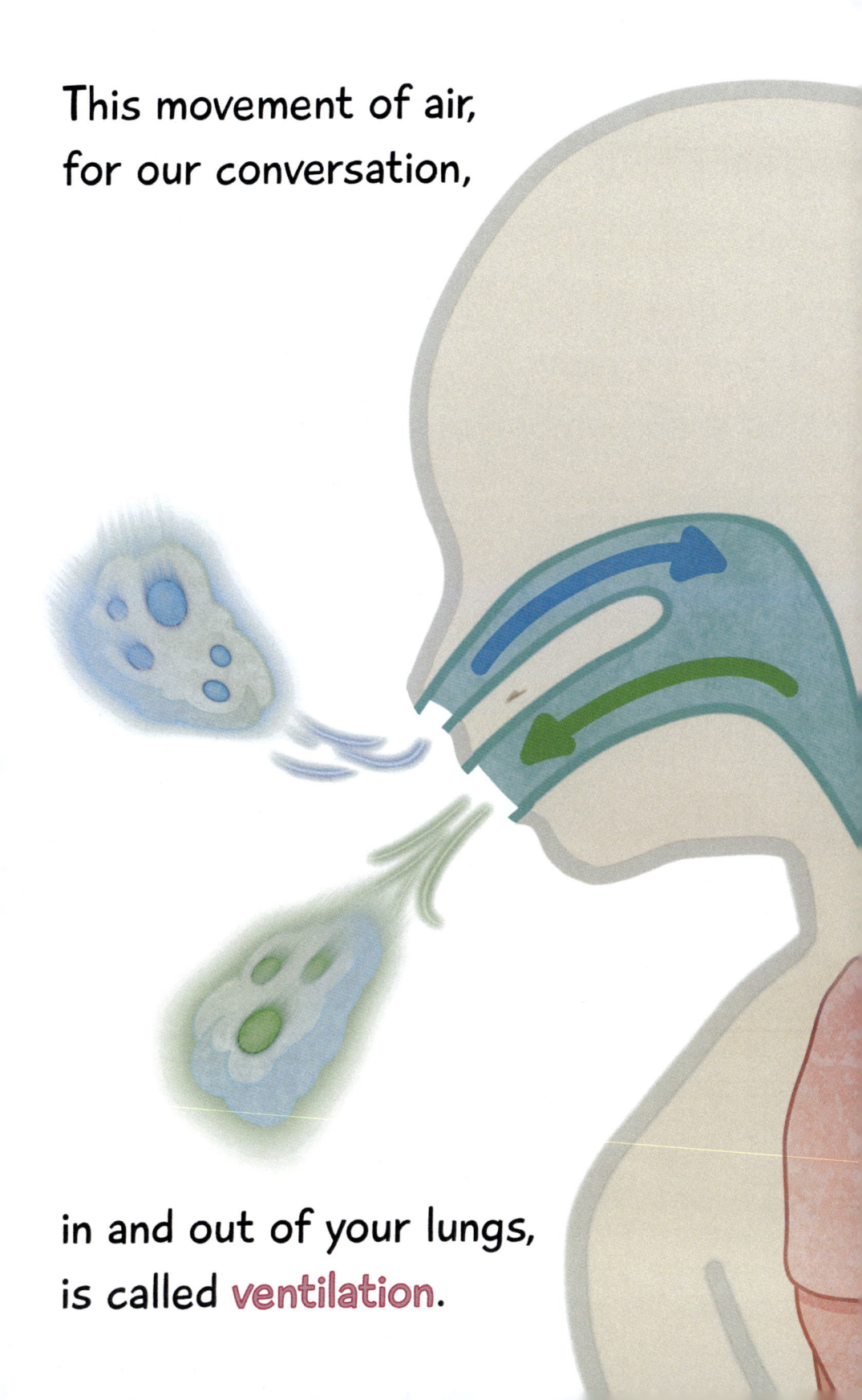

in and out of your lungs, is called ventilation.

Well, that's just about it.
That's how it gets done.

Inhale oxygen—
it's step number one.

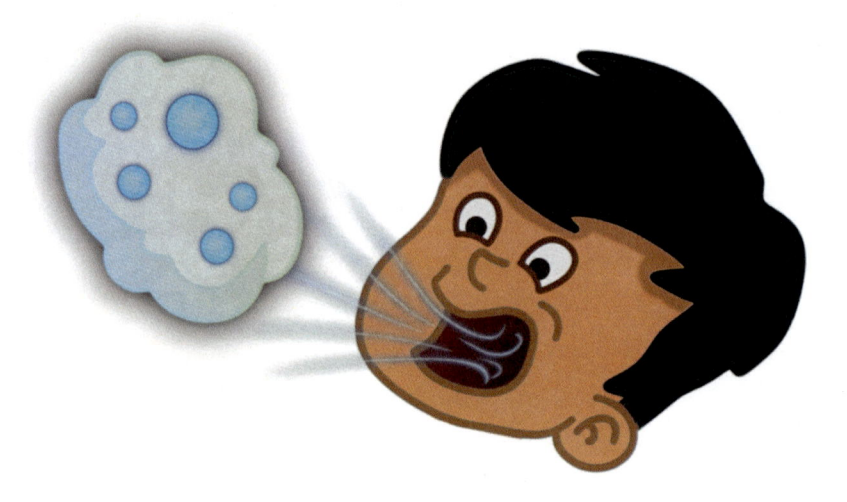

Energy gets made,
carbon dioxide produced,

then exhale it out.
Now you've been introduced

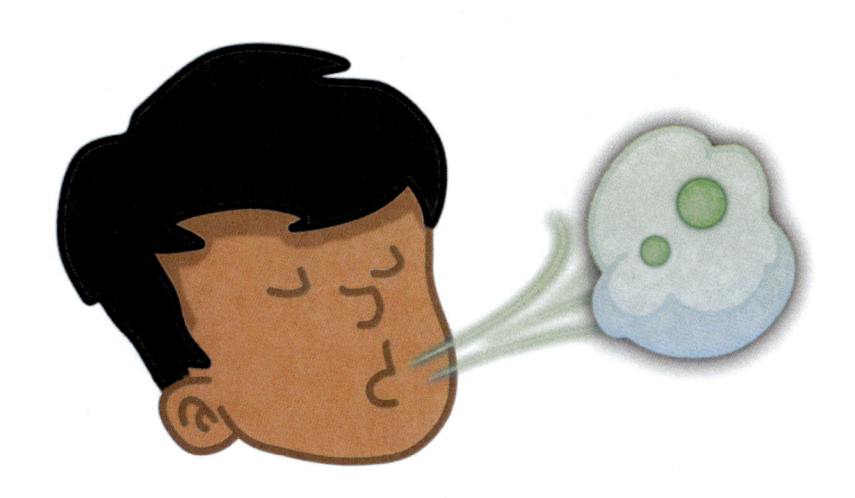

to the network of airways
and your breathing rhythm.

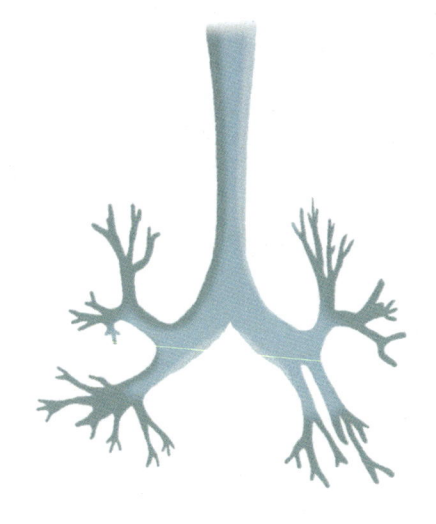

All together it's called...

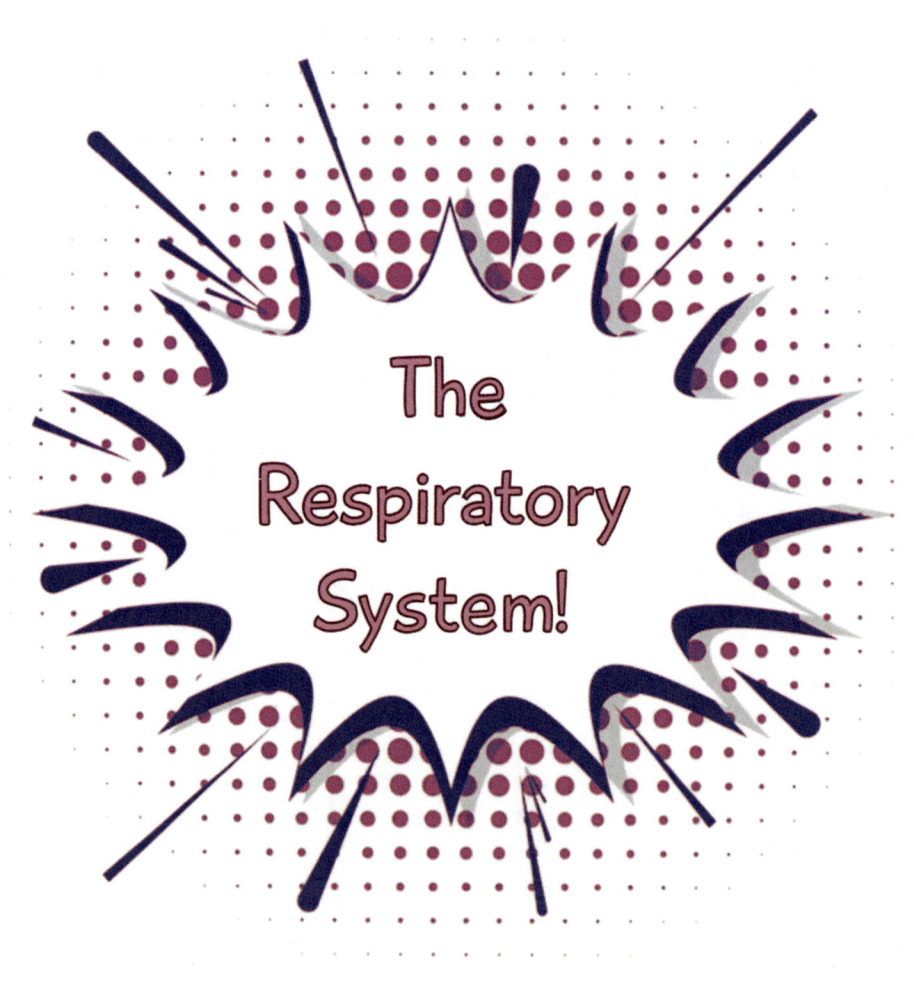

The Respiratory System!

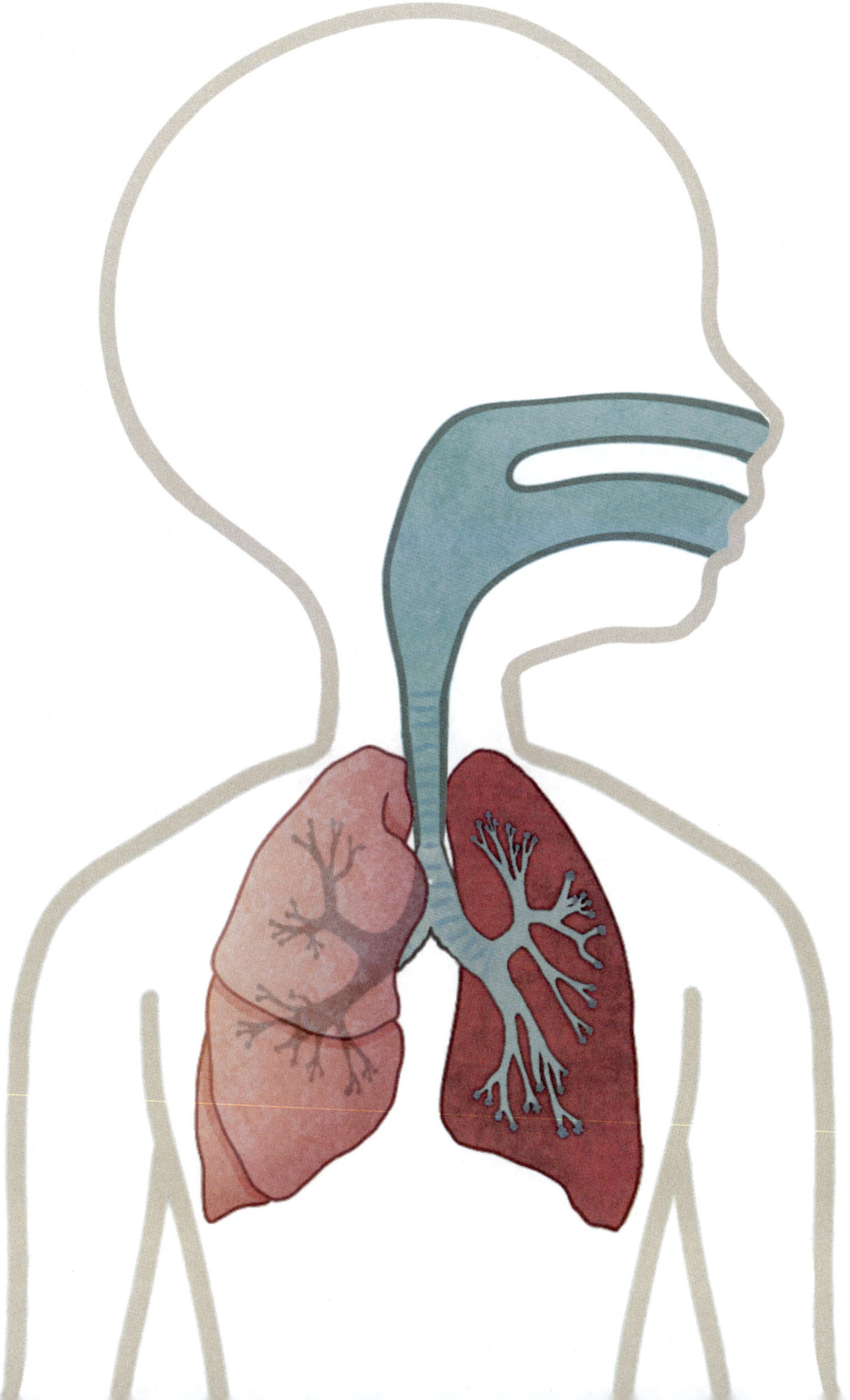

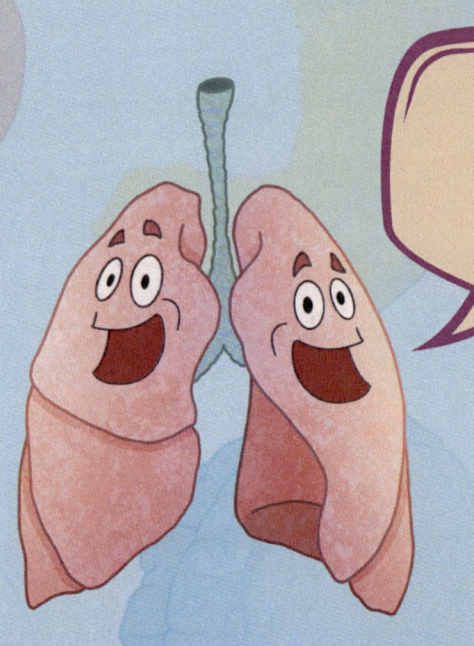

> Want to know more? Enjoy this bonus page and visit us at our website.

Tips for Healthy Lungs

- Improve your lung function with <u>regular physical activity</u>. Even a brisk walk will do.

- <u>Wash your hands</u> to help prevent respiratory infections like the cold, the flu, or pneumonia.

- <u>Avoid smoking, secondhand smoke, and vaping.</u> These can damage your lungs and lead to chronic lung disease or cancer.

- Sing out loud! <u>Singing can increase your lung capacity over time</u>, strengthen your respiratory muscles and even boost your mood.

More about the Respiratory System

- <u>Breathing in through your nose is best</u> because it warms, filters and humidifies the air.

- <u>Your left lung is smaller than your right lung</u> so it can make room in your chest for your heart.

- You learned WHY we breathe but what about HOW? When the muscle sitting under your lungs called <u>the diaphragm</u> contracts, air rushes in. When it relaxes, air gets pushed out.

- <u>The epiglottis</u> covers your trachea when you swallow to prevent food/water "going down the wrong pipe".

Fun Facts

- A doctor who takes care of lungs is called a <u>Pulmonologist</u>.

- Most of the air you breathe in isn't oxygen. It's 78% nitrogen, 21% oxygen and a tiny amount of argon, carbon dioxide, and other gasses.

- The surface area of all the alveoli in your lungs (about 600-800 square feet) is almost the size of an entire pickle ball court.

- You exhale a surprising amount of water every time you breathe out, totaling about 3 cups each day.

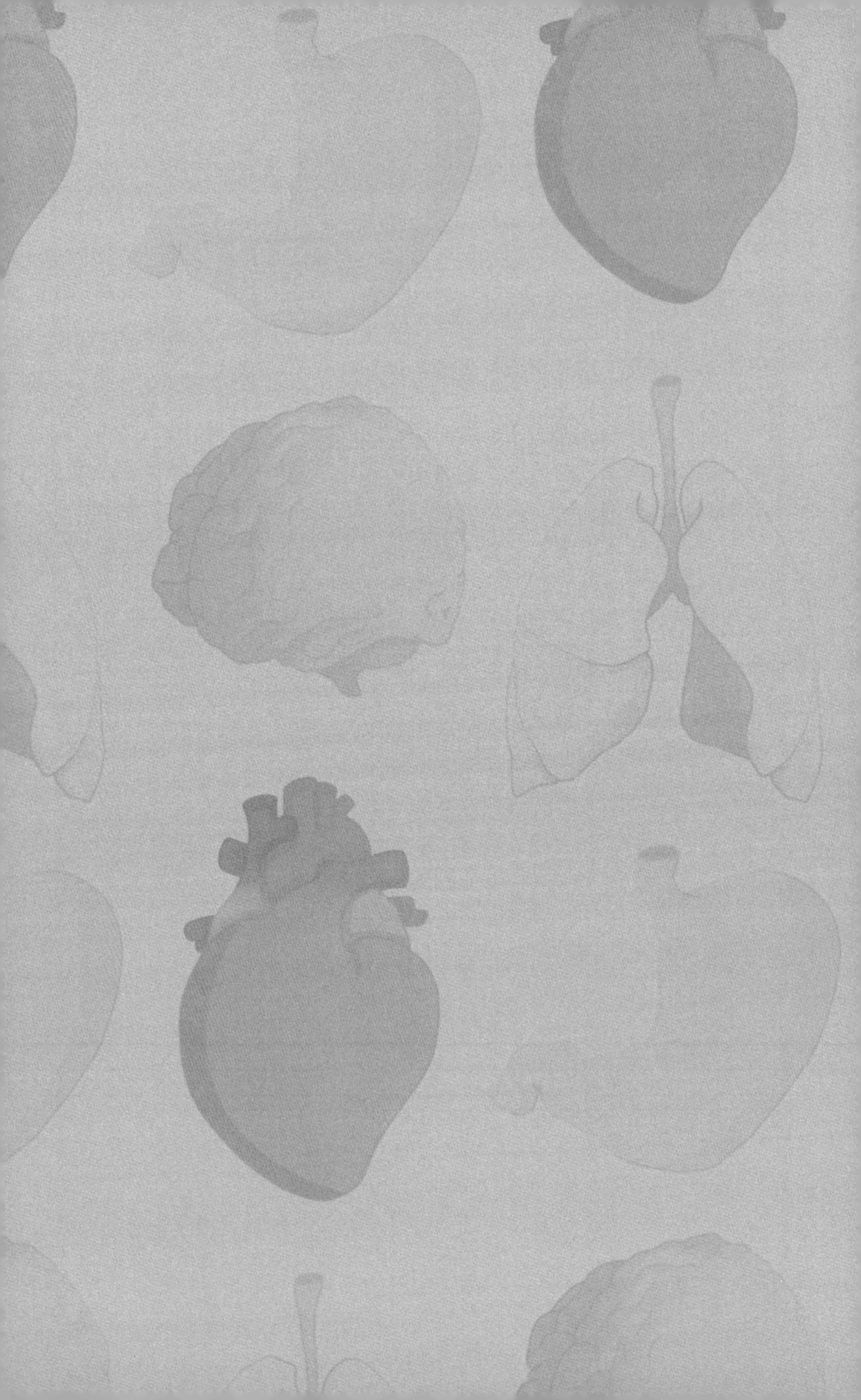

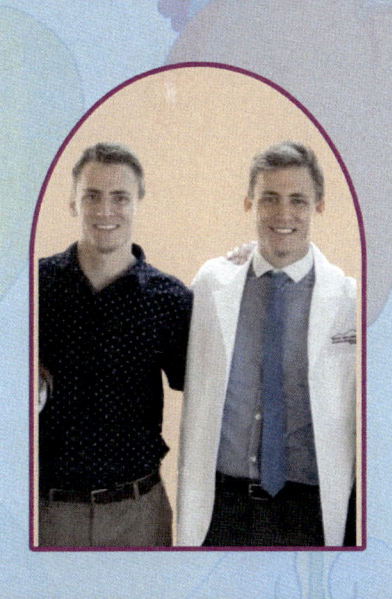

About the Author & Illustrator

As the saying goes, "two heads are better than one." That was never more apparent than when Bradley and Quintin were growing up. The McCann twins were often found working on various creative projects. Though inseparable during their upbringing, they each began their separate paths when Quintin accepted his first teaching job and Bradley applied to medical school. Years later, with the inception of Body McCannics, their paths merged again. Your Lungs, the second book in a short children's series about the human body, continues the ultimate collaboration for this doctor and artist duo.

Dedicated to Maeve,
who loves singing at the top of her lungs.

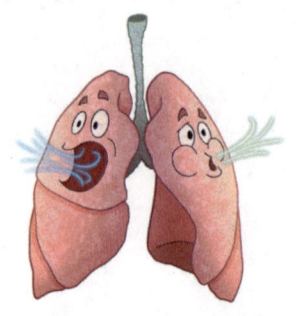

No part of this publication may be reproduced, stored in a retrieval system, or transmitted in any form or by any means, electronic, mechanical, photocopying, recording, or otherwise without written permission of the publisher.
First Body McCannics printing, November 2024.

Your Lungs, characters, text, and illustrations copyright © 2024 by Body McCannics. All rights reserved.
Published by Body McCannics.

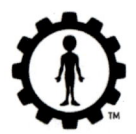

ISBN: 979-8-9913422-3-0

Library of Congress Control Number: 2024924253

For more learning, books, and games visit us here:

Made in the USA
Las Vegas, NV
15 February 2025